Acid Body: How to Eliminate an Acid Body

"If you are sick, the first thing to do is get rid of your acid body"

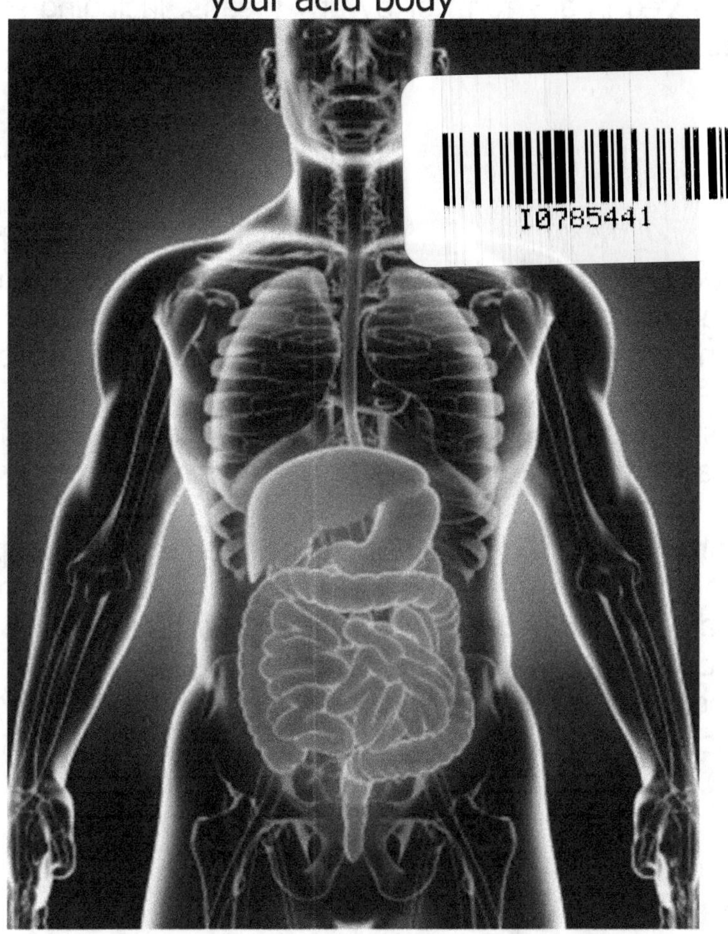

By Rudy S. Silva, Natural Nutritionist

Acid Body: How to Eliminate an Acid body "If you are sick, the first thing to do is get rid of your acid body" © 2018 by Rudy S. Silva

Disclaimer and Terms of Use: The Author and Publisher have strived to be as accurate and complete as possible in the creation of this book, notwithstanding the fact that he does not warrant or represent at any time that the contents within are accurate due to the rapidly changing nature of the Internet. While all attempts have been made to verify information provided in this publication, the Author and Publisher assume no responsibility for errors, omissions, or contrary interpretation of the subject matter herein.

Any perceived slights of specific persons, peoples, or organizations are unintentional. This book is not intended for use as a source of legal, business, accounting health, or financial advice. All readers are advised to seek services of competent professionals in legal, business, accounting, medical and finance field.

Printed 2018 in the United States of America

Table of Contents

1: Why an Acid Body is Dangerous

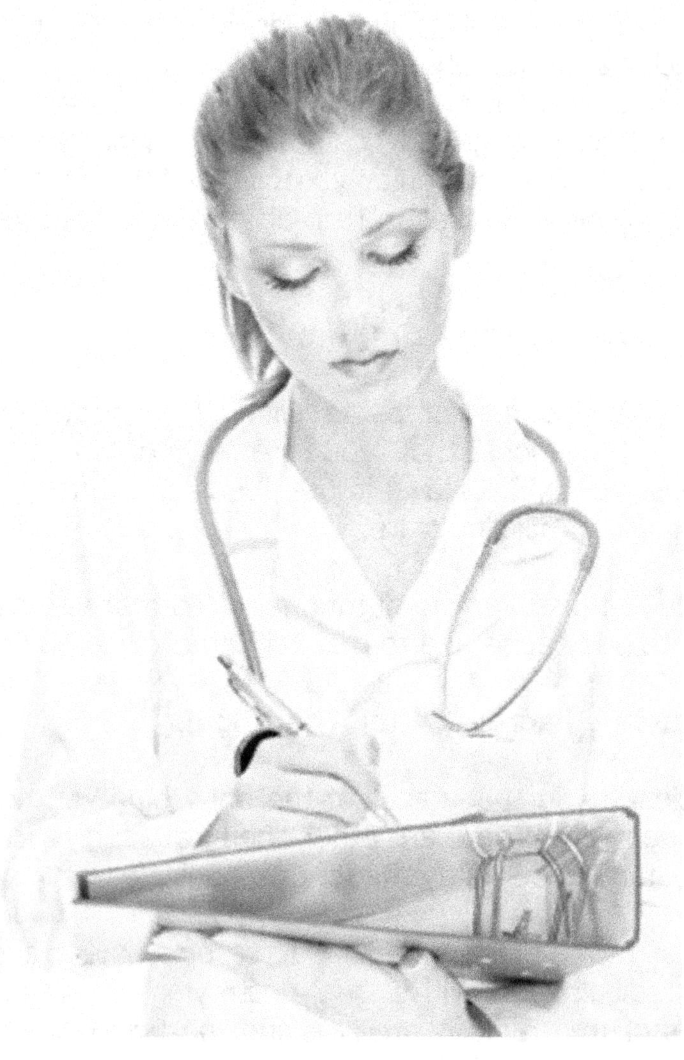

Acids in Your Body

Acids in your body are a major detriment to your health. If you can't diminish the level of body acids, you will not have decent health.

An acid body is a disease state. When you have a disease of any kind, the level of body acids is high. The higher your body acids are the more severe the illness.
An acid body attracts bacteria, pathogen, viruses, and other unwanted organisms. It creates an environment where disease can form and multiply. It is for this reason that you must know what it takes to turn an acid body into an alkaline body.

Steps to Change an Acid Body

One of the first steps in eliminating body acids is to examine the foods that you are eating. In the coming chapters, you will discover those foods that push your body into an acid or alkaline state.

You will discover the nutritional ideas that you can use to eliminate body acids and to maintain an alkaline body.

Destructive Factors Other Than Acids

Acids in your body are not the only thing you need to be concerned with. There are other chemicals and reactions that are created in your body that create acids.

Free radicals are a major source of sickness and illness. These radicals react with tissue, destroying its integrity. Some sources of free radicals are smoking, pesticides in food, food additives, air pollution, processed foods and contaminated water.

Personal Products

Personal products that you use on your body are filled with chemicals that lead to allergies, headaches, cardiovascular problems, and cancer; and the list goes on. No one really knows what the side effects personal products pose to each individual. What is known is that certain chemical found in personal products are detrimental to the health of many individuals, both in the short and long term.

Many of these products, soaps, creams, powders, toothpaste, create free radicals that become destructive.

In this book, you will discover what you need to know so that you don't become a victim of a terminal disease. Applying a few of these nutritional principles will give you the edge you need to create a body that can resist disease.

Acid Body

An acid body is where you have more acid in your body than your body can neutralize. When this happens, minerals that can neutralize these acids are pulled out of your hair, bile, organs, bones, lymph liquid and from other body locations. The body does this in an effort to prevent you from creating disease or dying. However, if these minerals are not supplied from your diet, your body will decay and die.

As your body decays from lack of minerals and the proper nutrition, there comes a point where cells, tissue or organs are no longer salvageable. That's the point where you need a new heart, kidney, liver, foot, leg, lung, and so on. That's the point where you have stage IV cancer.

This book is about how to stop your body's acids from destroying cells, tissue, organs, and body systems. It is also about how to stop the pain that goes with this acid destruction. There are many painful diseases associated with an acid body: Hiatus Hernia, Gout, Acid Reflux, Kidney stones, gallstones, etc.

There is only one way to stop acid, from destroying your body, and this is what you will learn in this book.

Acid Burning Foods and Concepts

To get rid of acids in your body, you need to eat certain fruits, vegetables, herbs, and supplements. Once this acid is neutralized, it is routed out of your body through your elimination channels.

You will be given a list of the best fruits and vegetables to eat that eliminate acids.

Body Cycles

There are three body cycles that you have. In the first body cycle, you will discover how to detoxify your body acids every morning.

The second and third cycle involves what you have to eat for lunch and dinner. These two cycles will not be covered. The first cycle is the most important since it's during this cycle that you take the most minerals for neutralizing your acids. In addition, the first body cycle is where your body is in a detoxification mode and you can help your body do just that.

The Power of Fruits

In the next chapters, you will discover more of why fruits have to the power to cure you, and drugs don't.

These chapters cover the importance of eating and using fruits and vegetables and other nutrients to keep healthy and to recover from sickness. Fruits and vegetables are central, to neutralizing acids and creating an alkaline body. There are some fruits that are considered acid and some that are alkaline. You will discover what this really means, and how your body uses these different types of produce to create a body with a strong immune system.

2: Use Litmus Paper to Identify an Acid Body

Measuring Your Body's Acids

In this chapter, you will learn how to measure your saliva and urine to determine the level of acid in your body. Using pH litmus paper, you can measure your initial acid body condition and then continue to monitor it, as you apply the changes recommended, in this book.

With litmus pH paper, you can measure your saliva and urine. Using these readings, you can start making changes, in your eating habits and lifestyle. Then you can re-measure your saliva and urine, to see what improvements you have made towards eliminating an acid body and creating an alkaline body.

Using litmus paper to monitor your health is a super idea. If you are not inclined to do this, get someone else to help you or to partner up with.

Checking your own acid level is great way to commit to taking control of your health. You will have a reading that will motivate you to keep changing your diet.

If your pH tests show that your body's acids are high, this means that your alkaline reserves are low. You will be changing some eating habits so that you increase your alkaline reserves. A high alkaline reserve indicates that you can neutralize acids and still have reserves left over.

Where to buy pH Litmus Paper

The first thing you want to do is buy pH litmus paper that gives you accurate readings. Buy the paper that comes in pH increments of 0.2 or 0.25.

You can purchase some pH litmus paper at a drug store, laboratory outlet or through the Internet. Go to Amazon and get this product, PHion Balance Diagnostic pH Test Strips, .25 increments. This is the easiest way to get this pH paper.

Three Days of Testing

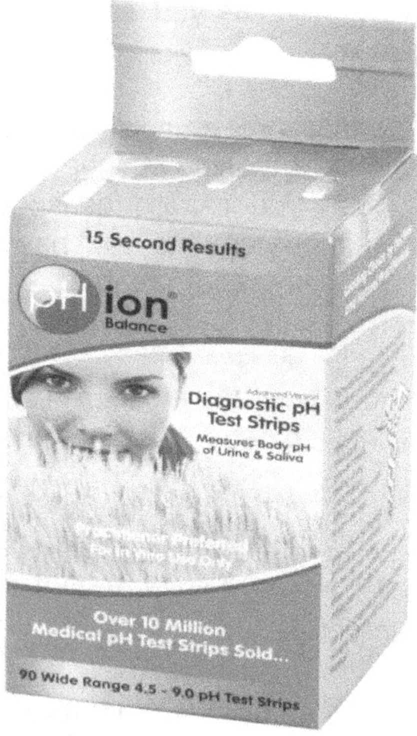

You need to take these pH tests for three days and for at least two to three times a day to get an average value. This will establish a pH baseline or a starting health point for you.

You will be doing these tests, as you progress through these outlined steps. This will evaluate how you are doing in this program. These tests are not exact clinical tests, but they are good enough for checking your body's acid levels as you progress through this program.

The three pH tests to do are:

- pH saliva test

- Lemon pH saliva test

- urine test

Saliva Test

Here is a simple test you can perform on your saliva that will give you an idea of where you stand with your body pH level. Your saliva contains mineral salts that keep it alkaline at 6.8 to 7.4. If your body is deficient in minerals, it will take the minerals from your saliva causing it to drop in pH, which means it is more acidic.

If your saliva is below 6.8 to 7.2 (normal readings), you can influence your saliva's pH to read higher, by eating more acid binding (acid binding food will be explained in the next chapter) food and to supplement with potassium, magnesium, and calcium.

You need to take this test for 3 days and at least 2 to 3 times a day and get an average value so that you can establish a baseline or a starting point for yourself.

Starting Your Saliva Testing

Gather saliva in your mouth then swallow. Do this three to four times. Place the pH paper under your tongue. Let it sit there for 5 seconds to wet it.

Now, remove it from your mouth. Let it sit for 10 seconds, compare the color of your pH paper to the color chart on the bottle and record the pH.

Do this test around one hour before eating or around two hours after eating. This reading gives you an idea about the state of your saliva. Your first test should be done first thing in the morning before you rinse out your mouth or drink anything.

Saliva and Lemon Test

Now, do this test immediately after you do your saliva test above. Squeeze half of the lemon juice in one ounce of water and swish it around in your mouth for 5 seconds or so then spit it out, wait one minute, now, measure your mouth's pH with litmus paper. Just place the paper into your mouth and wet it.

Now, compare the color and pH value of this reading with your first pH saliva reading. This reading should have a higher alkaline reading than your first saliva reading.

Good Saliva Test

If this reading has a higher alkaline reading, it means you have alkaline reserves. The higher the alkaline reading you have the stronger your alkaline reserves. A small alkaline upward change means you have alkaline reserves, but they are not as strong as they should be.

For example,

- Morning reading is 6.5 pH (the higher the better)
- After the lemon test reading 6.9 pH

These readings are good and indicate you have somebody mineral stores. But, your Morning reading of 6.5 is a little low and should be closer to 7.0 for better health.

Weak Saliva Test

If your pH reading does not change from your first reading or actually goes down by becoming more acidic, then your alkaline reserves are weak, and you need to make some major changes in the way you eat. In this course, you will see what you will need to do to bring up your alkaline reserves so that you will not be susceptible to serious diseases.

Now, suppose your readings were,

- First reading 6.5
- Lemon test reading 6.2

There is a drop in your lemon pH, and this is not too good. This means that you don't have enough minerals in your body to neutralize the acid in your mouth. You will have to eat more acid binding food.

Saliva Test Summary

Again, if your lemon test readings have a higher pH reading than your first reading, it means you have alkaline reserves. The bigger the difference between your first test and second test, the stronger your alkaline reserves. A small alkaline upward change means you have alkaline reserves, but they are not as strong as they should be.

If your lemon pH reading does not change from your first reading or actually goes down by becoming more acidic, then your alkaline reserves are weak, and you need to make some major changes in the way you eat. This also means you have a highly acidic body that can create some serious illness, especially if your lemon test pH is down to 6.0 and below.

Urine pH test

There have been clinical studies indicating that urine pH is an accurate reflection of your body responding to the production of acid waste.

Each time you test your urine, note what you ate in the previous evening meal. Eating a high-protein meal, which is an acid meal, will require more acid binding minerals to neutralize your acid dinner. If you eat a meal high in vegetables and little protein, then your body should easily neutralize your meal by morning.

Here's how to do the urine pH test

In the morning when you first urinate, allow it to flow for a second and then wet your pH litmus paper with urine.

If your urine pH is below 6.0 or 5.8, this indicates that your body did not have enough alkaline ash or ions to neutralize your evening dinner. In addition, you do not have enough alkaline mineral reserves to protect your body from acid damage to your cells and tissues.

If your urine is down to 5.8, this is on the low side but is considered ok. But, this is not a good place for your pH to be at all the times. You want your urine pH to be close to 6.5. This shows that you have plenty of mineral stores to neutralize the previous night's acid dinner – meat or carbohydrates.

Normal Urine Range is 5.8 to 6.5

A good urine range is from 6.0 and 6.5, indicating that your alkaline reserves are in good shape. Of course, the closer you are to 6.5, the better and this is the pH you should strive for.

High Urine pH

If your morning urine is over 7.2 and higher, this indicates your body is going into an emergency state, using ammonia from the liver in an effort to reduce your body's acids. You may read as high as 8.0 indicating for sure you are producing ammonia to neutralize your acid dinner. To change this will require a substantial change in your eating habits. Sometimes you can smell that your urine is ammonia-like.

Keep in mind that this may be temporary, but if you consistently see high urine pH, then you definitely have a problem and need to back off from eating acid food.

Test Your Urine for 3 days

Test your urine for 3 days to see if it remains consistent. Record this information to see how it changes as you progress through this program.

- Measure your saliva pH in the morning.

- Measure your morning urine

- Measure your urine pH two times during the day.

- Measure your urine mid-day, two hours after eating

If your initial pH tests indicate that you have an acid body, then depending on how acidic it is this will determine how long you have work to change your body's acid levels.

Compute the pH Average

After three or four days of saliva and urine readings, you want to take the average of all readings. Here is how you can determine what your pH readings mean.

- pH level of 6.5 to 7.4 - You are at a healthy level. However, the higher number is better.

- pH level of 6.0 to 6.5 – You may not be feeling good and need to make some changes in your diet.

- pH level of 5.0 to 6.0 - You have major health problems.

- pH level of 4.5 – 5.0 – You have a terminal disease.

You are considered to have an alkaline body if your overall body pH liquids are 6.5 to 7.4. This is the pH level that you should strive for. Higher pH values of 7.5 to 8.5 and up are considered detrimental.

Children with an acid body will respond quickly to good changes in eating habits, whereas adults, depending on age, can see results in 5 weeks and up to a year.

A pH Guide

Here is a guideline to what your saliva and urine pH should be.

- Saliva should be 6.6 to 7.4
- Urine should be 5.8 to 6.4

If your urine is down to 5.8, this is ok, since it shows that you are getting rid of body acids. But, you don't always want to have such a low reading. For saliva, a good reading is 6.8.

3: Minerals, the Secret to Burning Acids

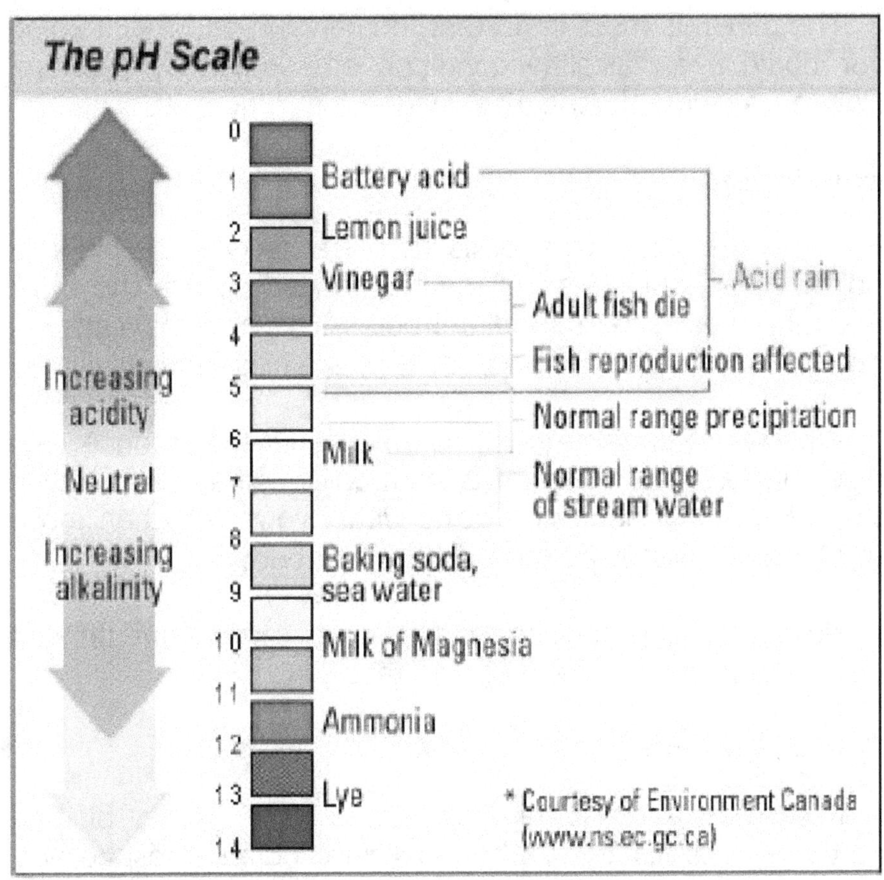

Minerals

Making your body more alkaline is what will give you the best curative effects of fruits, vegetable, and supplements. An alkaline body prevents your body from becoming ill and forming deadly diseases, like joint problems, organ degradation, body pain, or even cancer.

If you are already sick, then all the chemicals inside fruits will help to revive you to better health. This is provided that your tissue damage has not gone beyond repair.

The minerals most important in changing and maintaining your body in an alkaline condition are sodium, potassium, chloride, calcium, phosphorus, magnesium, and sulfur.

Acid Binding

There are certain minerals that are called acid binding. And these are minerals, as mentioned earlier, are the most important ones in fruits, Sodium, potassium, chloride, calcium, phosphorus, magnesium because they are acid binding.

What acid binding means is when you eat produce with these minerals, your cells, after metabolism, create an alkaline ash. This ash will neutralize acids within your cells then move out of your cells to seek out acids in your body.

Now, these neutralized acids will be carried out of your body through your urine, bile, and feces. T

Alkaline Binding

Now, there are also minerals that become alkaline binding and these minerals are sulphur, chlorine, iodine, phosphorous, bromine, fluorine, copper, and silicon.

It is these minerals that when digested by a cell will produce an acid salt that will bind with alkaline minerals. These minerals will be excreted through your urine. When alkaline minerals are bonded to an acid salt, the alkaline mineral is removed from your body, and your body becomes more acidic, the condition you are trying to avoid.

4: The Best Fruits-Vegetables that Neutralize Acids

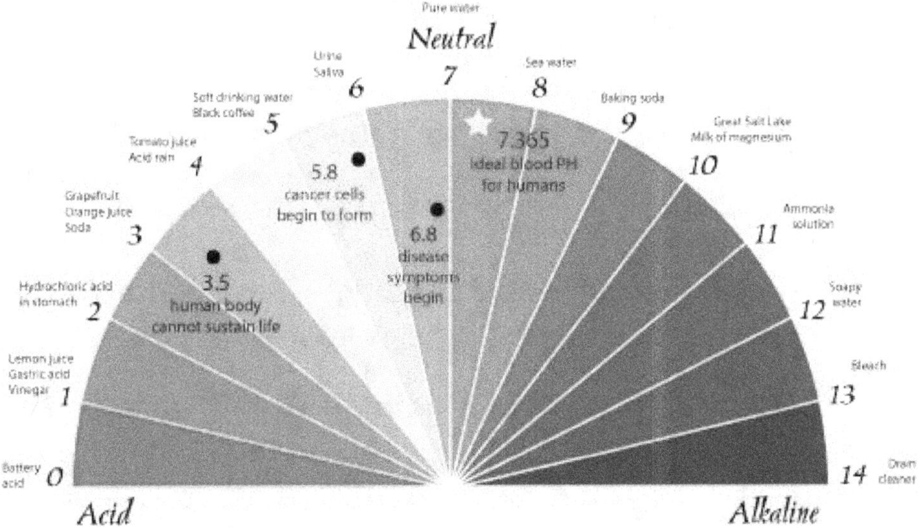

Acid Binding Fruits and Vegetables

Here is a list of fruits, vegetables and other foods that have the highest alkaline and acid minerals. The percentage number next to these foods indicates the strength of the alkaline minerals or acid minerals. The closer to 100% the more effective these foods are as an acid-reducing or an alkaline reducing food. However, you should be eating all foods throughout the list not just the ones at the top of the list.

The percentage assigned to these fruits is based on fresh fruits and vegetables that are organic and not cooked, canned or mixed with sugar. If they are cooked or otherwise processed in some fashion, this will slightly reduce their effectiveness as an acid binding. However, they will still be effective in acid binding.

Acid Binding Fruits with Alkaline Minerals

To create an alkaline body, you need to eat 80% acid binding food and 20% alkaline binding food. Work towards this end and you will slowly make your body more acid to alkaline.

Here is the list of foods to eat in the order of priority.

Fruits

1. **Fruits at 100% Acid Binding – Best fruits To Eat**
   Lemons, melons – any type, watermelon

2. **Fruits at 93% Acid Binding – Great fruits To Eat**
   Cantaloupes, dried dates, dried figs, limes, mango, papaya

3. **Fruits at 87% Acid Binding – Still Great Fruits To Eat**
   Kiwis, passion fruit, pineapples, raisins, umeboshi plums

4. **Fruits at 80% Acid Binding – Eat These Fruits**
   Apricots, avocados, bananas, fresh dates, fresh figs, currants, gooseberries grapes, grapefruits guavas, kumquats, nectarines, pears, persimmons, quince, berries, cactus

5. **Fruits at 73% Acid Binding – Still Fruits To Eat**
   Apples, oranges, peaches, pomegranate, raspberries, sour grapes, strawberries, carob

6. **Fruits at 67% Acid Binding – Still Neutralizes Acids** Cherries, fresh coconut

7. **Herbal Teas From Leaves at 73% to 86% acid binding**

Alfalfa, mint, sage, spearmint, raspberry strawberry comfrey

8. **All Herbs and Spices** at 67% to 73% Acid Binding

9. **Fruits** At 40% to 47%   - Eat less of these fruits
   Blueberries, cranberries, plums, prunes

10. **All Fruit Juices** From A Juicer 100% Acid Binding

Vegetables

Here is the list of vegetables to eat in order of priority. All of these vegetables will neutralize acid, since they contain minerals that are acid binding.

1. Vegetables at 93% Acid Binding – best vegetables to eat
   Kelp, Seaweed, Watercress, Asparagus

2. Vegetables at 80% Acid Binding – Still the best to eat
   Lettuce Leaf, Oyster plant, Pumpkin, Spinach, Squash, Peas, Carrots, Celery, Chard, Swiss, Dandelion greens

3. Vegetables at 73% Acid Binding – Great vegetables to eat
   Bamboo shoots, Beets, Broccoli, Cabbage, Cauliflower, Collards, Corn, sweet, Ginger (fresh), Mushrooms, Mustard greens, Onions, Pepper, Potatoes, Green, Lima, String, Potatoes

4. Vegetables at 67% Acid Binding – eat plenty of these Brussell sprouts, Cucumbers, Eggplant, Okra, Onions, Radishes, Tomatoes

5. Vegetable juices at 80% to 93% Acid Binding Parsley, wheatgrass, carrot, celery, etc.

6. Soy Bean Products at 60% Acid Binding – limit your use of tofu since it is a genetically modified organism, MO Dried beans, Soy cheese, Soy milk, Tempeh, Tofu

7. Here are some other misc. foods to eat that are acid binding.

8. Starches at 80% Acid Binding
Arrowroot flour

9. Sugar at 73% acid Binding
Honey

10. Nuts and Seeds at 60 % to 67% Acid Binding Almonds, sesame seeds, Granola, Essene Bread, Chestnuts

11. Misc. foods at 60% Acid Binding
Horseradish, Amaranth, Millet, Quinoa, Dried beans, Soy cheese, Soy milk,

The following foods are alkaline binding, which means that they create acids that will bind with alkaline salts and remove them from your body. These foods when eaten in excess will create an acid body. You should only eat around 20% of these foods in your diet, and the other 80% should come from fruits and vegetables or foods that are acid binding. When you eat with this 80/20 formula, you will have an alkaline body.

NOTE: The lower the alkaline binding percentage, the more that food is acid producing.

1. **All oils are basically at 50% and are considered neutral.**

   This includes almond, avocado, canola, coconut, corn castor, olive, soy, sunflower oil, and etc.

2. **Beans, starches, and nuts and seeds at 40% to 46% Alkaline Binding**

   Aduki, Black, Broadbean, Garbanzo, Mung, Pinto, Barley, Corn Meal, Lentils, Brans, Cashews, Coconut (dried), Pecans, Brans, Millet, Filberts, Walnuts, Pumpkin, Sunflower

3. **Starches at 26 to 33 % Alkaline Binding**

   Brown Rice, Buckwheat, Oats, Spelt, Wheat Whole, Peanuts, corn, rye

4. **Rice at 20% Alkaline Binding**

   White rice

5. **Sugar at 13% Alkaline Binding**

   White beet or cane sugar

6. **Meat and Fish**

7. **Meat at 26% alkaline binding**

   Fish With fins and scales, Shellfish - shrimp, scallops, crab lobster, oyster

8. **Meat at 20% Alkaline Binding**

   Chicken, turkey, rabbit

9. **Meat at 13% Alkaline Binding**

   Beef, goat, pork, lamb

11. **All oils are basically at 50% and are considered neutral**.

    This includes almond, avocado, canola, coconut, corn castor, olive, soy, sunflower oil, and etc.

12. **Misc. Products at 13% to 26% Alkaline Binding**

    Liquor, wine, beer, coffee, black tea, caffeine drinks

5: Use Body Cycle 1 to Flush out Acids Daily

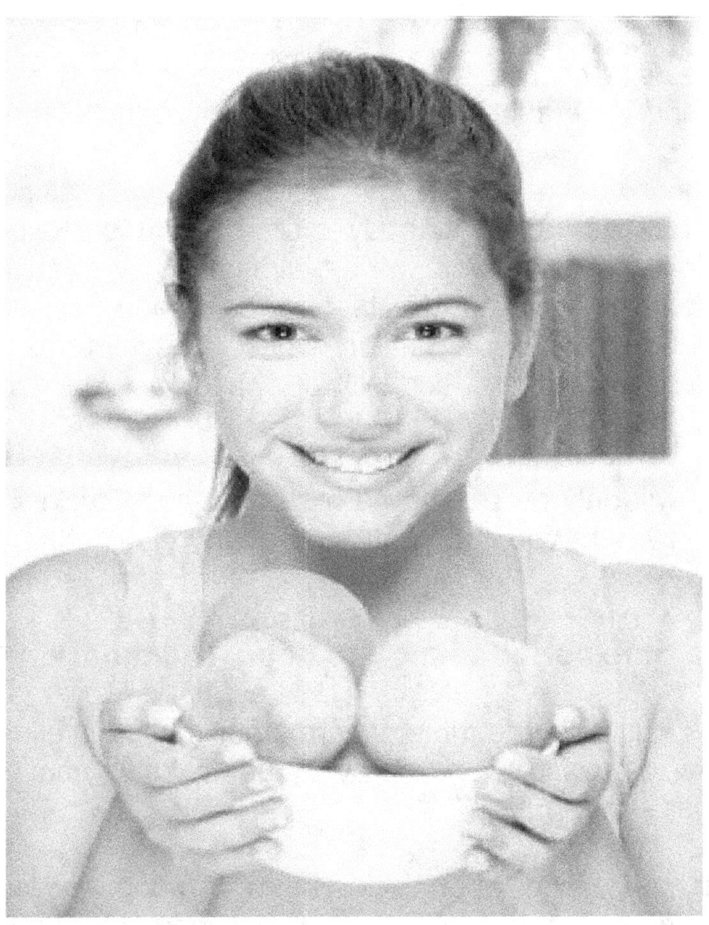

Natural Body Cycles

Most of you are looking for ways to improve your health, lose weight, or get rid of an illness that you have. Here's some information that will help you achieve these results. It is called "Using Your Natural Body Cycles" for achieving maximum health. Getting in tune with your Natural Body Cycles requires a change in the way you eat.

Since all of us are addicted to the way we eat, it is sometimes difficult to change these habits. But, if you are serious about what you want, this is the best information that will give you good health.

Here is a chance to use the information in the chapter "Fruits And Vegetable That Neutralize Body Acids"

Using your natural body cycles, you will gain better health. But, as you apply body cycles, you might experience side effects, because you will be eliminating body toxins and body wastes. The side effects may be headaches, stomach upsets, body pain, or similar types of symptoms. These conditions will not last and will disappear as you get rid of more toxins.

You will only be concerned here with body cycle 1. Body cycle 1 is where you can gain the most by eliminating an acid body.

Cycle 1 time period: 4 a.m. to noon (Elimination Cycle)

This cycle is the time where your body is eliminating toxins, acids, wastes, and derby by urine, bowel movements, and other secretions.

During the elimination cycle, 4 a.m. to noon, eat and drink only fruits and their juices or drink vegetable juices. For breakfast eat a bowl of fruit or have a fruit smoothie made with apple juice and fruits in season. Before noontime eat fruits as a snack. Forty-five minutes before noon eat your last fruit. You can eat and drink all the fruits and juices you want up to noontime.

By eating in this way you are assisting your body's elimination cycle. This helps your body to eliminate toxins and acids from your body and blood. It is these toxins and acids that make you sick and overweight. Acids are the main cause of most illnesses, and so you want to have an alkaline body. Fruits and vegetables give you an alkaline body.

It takes 1 hour or so to digest fruit and fruit juices. Because of this, they help to cleanse your body of waste. Fruits are 70% water just like your body, and this gives them the cleansing action that your body needs.

Eating a typical breakfast of eggs, potatoes, meat, bacon, bread, butter, and jelly, interferes with your elimination cycle. These foods required 3 to 4 hours to digest, so your body gets busy digesting these foods instead of detoxifying your body with fruits and juices.

Cycle 2 time period: noon to 8 p.m.

This is the time when your body should be taking in food and digesting. During this period, is the time to eat solid food. What you eat has to be in alignment with what your stomach can do.

Cycle 3 time period: 8 p.m. to 4 a.m.

This is the time your body is absorbing and using the food you have eaten during the 12 noon to 8 p.m. period. This is the time the food you have eaten during the day is assimilated, absorbed and distributed throughout your body through your blood.

To learn more about body cycles 2 and 3, they are detailed completely in the book called "body Alkaline Body."

6: How Fruits Fix Your Acid Body

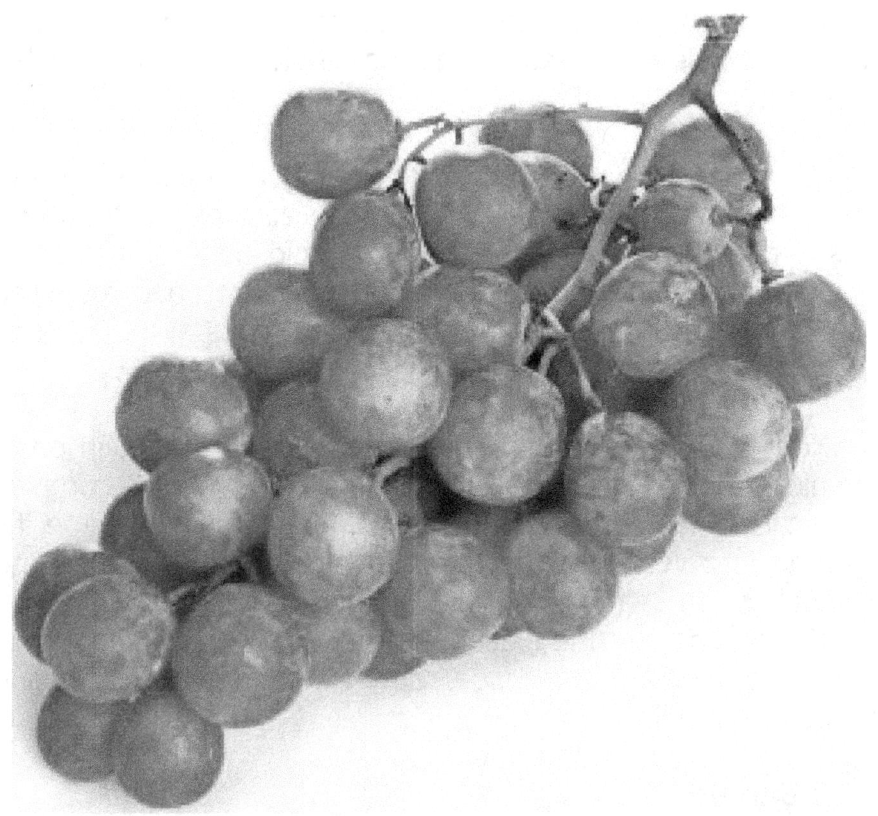

Because fruits are naturally grown from the soil, they pull minerals from the ground and can be a great source of nutrients for you, if the soil is heavy with minerals. Because of these minerals and other nutrients, Fruits have amazing curative effects, when they are eaten raw. In some cases, it is better to cook them for their healing effects.

The best fruits to eat are those that allow your body to become more alkaline. Your body naturally seeks to be in an alkaline condition. In this condition, your body has less pain, inflammation, and disease. It has more energy, and your body is not deteriorating as fast as when your body is filled with acid.

It's ok to eat fruits that make your body acid. However, eating more fruits that make your body alkaline is necessary. This is because most people have an acid body and need to move it to an alkaline condition. Later when you become more alkaline, you will be eating 80% alkaline fruits and 20% acid fruits.

Your body uses minerals to neutralize acids and, in other chemical body reactions, to create simple or complex chemicals that your body needs. So, the body holds specific minerals in a certain way. It holds minerals in "storage" and releases them when they are needed for certain chemical reactions. The storage locations of minerals are in the blood, in organs, in cells, in tissue, and in the liquid inside and outside your cells.

Fruit Benefits

Fruits contain a variety of nutrients that are necessary for maintaining life. Each nutrient has its function in the body. Many of the functions are known, and many are not. Here is a list of some of the main known nutrients and what they do in your body.

Minerals
Antioxidants
Vitamins
Fiber
Natural water

Enzymes
Phytonutrients
Unknown chemicals

Minerals

Your body contains around 4% minerals by weight.

Minerals have a lot of functions in the body. Your body's growth and development depend on minerals. They act as partners with enzymes to work in your body to reduce inflammation. They provide structural support in bones and teeth, maintain water balance, are involved in muscle contraction and assist in enzyme function.

They combine with other molecules to form complex ions such as hemoglobin. They work to help **maintain alkaline-acid balance** throughout your entire body. And, they assist in the transmission of information from the brain to all body systems.

You don't hear your mother saying, "take your minerals," normally you hear, "don't forget to take your vitamins, or eat your vegetables." But, minerals are one step above vitamins in that many vitamins cannot do their job in your body without minerals.

There are two types of minerals. First, there are regular minerals such as calcium, sodium, phosphorous, magnesium, and potassium. These are the minerals you normally take daily.

Then there are trace minerals and these are like zinc, copper, arsenic, and iron. It's in the trace minerals that you can run the risk of mineral toxicity since you don't need much of these trace minerals. Of course, there are more minerals in each category. Here is a list of the major minerals you find in fruits.

Sodium, potassium, chloride, calcium, phosphorus, magnesium, manganese

Here is a list of the trace minerals:

Iron, selenium, zinc, copper, iodide, fluoride, chromium, molybdenum, boron, nickel, silicon, arsenic, vanadium

Minerals are found both in meat and in fruits and vegetables. Our concentration here is on minerals found in fruits and how they can cure your body. Most all minerals are found in fruits, but there are some that are only found in meat and other foods.

There are other minerals that are called heavy metals. These tend to displace other beneficial minerals and cause toxic effects. These metals are:

Lead, cadmium, mercury, arsenic, iron

Vitamins

Vitamins are needed in small amounts in your body to perform normal functions, to provide for growth and to assist in body maintenance. There are two types of vitamins, fat-soluble and water-soluble.

Most vitamins cannot be made in the body. Some can but in small amounts. For this reason, most vitamins that your body needs must come from the food you eat. Some fruits have vitamins, but they will not have all the vitamins your body needs.

Vitamins carry out various complex biochemical or physiological reactions in your body. When you lack the necessary vitamins your body needs, these chemical reactions do not occur often enough. The result is the creation of various illnesses. If the illnesses are not too far along, the illness can be reversed.

As with all illnesses, when it is not too far along, it can be reversed with the appropriate minerals, vitamins, or nutrients. In many cases, people wait too long before they address their illness. Sometimes, people don't know they are ill, or they just ignore that they don't feel good.

When an illness is reversible, then you need the foods that have the nutrients that will make you well and not the drugs that will keep or make you sick.

When you wait too long, when you have an illness, you get tissue damage in your organs, veins, arteries, or body that is not reversible using natural methods. Surgery or drugs can sometimes repair tissue damage, but you will not be the same as before when you were well.

Antioxidants

The body produces antioxidants to neutralize the free radicals that become excessive in your body. Free radicals have a damaging effect on the tissue they encounter as they float throughout your body. Left uncheck they cause numerous deadly diseases.

The way the body takes care of this threat is to create antioxidants. However, the body's antioxidants are not always enough to capture all the free radicals. This is because free radical can be created in numerous ways and can be found in food, air, water, and personal products.

Free radicals are also created by emotional states such as anger, fear, depression, and anxiety.

The result is that your body needs help to neutralize these free radicals, and this is where fruits come in. They are packed with antioxidants. Using them to neutralize free radicals has become a necessity.

There are many minerals and vitamins that are classified as antioxidants. These are vitamins A, C, E, and selenium. Other antioxidants are bioflavonoids, carotenoids, isoflavones, all minerals, allium vegetables like garlic and onions, bilberry, coenzyme Q10, cruciferous vegetables, ginkgo biloba, glutathione, lipoic acid, superoxide dismutase, and melatonin.

Antioxidants and Phytonutrients

Phytochemicals or phytonutrients are mostly found in the skin of fruits and are considered antioxidants. These nutrients give the fruit its color. Fruits also contain the fundamental antioxidants, vitamin A, C, E, beta-carotene, zinc, and selenium. Try to buy organic fruits so you can eat the skins without worry. In some fruits, there are more nutrients on the skin than in the fruit.

Other antioxidants that you may have heard of are carotenoids, lutein, lycopene, sod, and glutathione, anthocyanins, and lipoic acid. The list is in the hundreds.

Phytonutrients are special nutrients that are found in fruits and other plants. In plants, they protect them from disease, insects, excess heat, UV rays, poisons, pollutants, injury, and drought.

Phytonutrients have been found to be beneficial to human life. They contain chemicals that are useful in treating and preventing diseases such as cancer, diabetes, cardiovascular disease, and hypertension.

The phytonutrients consist of many groups, but the most important groups are the phytosterols and phytohormones. These sterols are precursors to your human sterols.

Bioflavonoids

Bioflavonoids are also antioxidants that are chemicals, which come from water-soluble colors found in fruits, vegetables, grains, leaves, and barks. Because they are found in a variety of plant foods, they come in different chemical forms and concentrations.

Some of the bioflavonoids are more powerful in destroying free radicals then the standbys, vitamin C and E. Some well-known flavonoids are catechins, resveratrol, and proanthocyanidins.

Enzymes

Enzymes are composed of different amino acids connected together. The body can create many enzymes, but not all, because it not all amino acids are created in the body. There are some amino acids that only come from the food you eat. So you need to eat certain foods to get the amino acids your body needs to create all the necessary enzymes.

Without enzyme activity in your body, you could not live. These chemical entities are required to help you breathe, give you energy, digest food, allow you to hear and see, and perform thousands of other body activities. There are over 75,000 of these enzymes in our body, and their chemical activity is constantly going on.

Enzymes are molecules that are catalysts. They start the chemical reaction of other molecules and compounds to produce the chemicals or functions that your body needs.

The body can only produce so many enzymes, and if you are sick, stressed, injured, depressed, or aged, then you will produce less. This will cause you to become even sicker.

You can also get enzymes from the raw food that you eat, which will supplement your body's enzymes. Enzymes are found in large quantities in raw fruits and vegetables. When food is processed and exposed to heat and encapsulated in a vacuum, the enzymes are destroyed.

All fruits have enzymes that help you digest them. This is why it is best to eat them raw so you can benefit from the natural enzymes. Eating fruits raw instead of cooked, in cans, in bottles, or in any other processed package saves your own body's enzymes.

Enzymes are usually destroyed at about 115 deg F. That is why raw fruits are better for you than cooked fruits.

Your body has only a certain number of enzymes that it can produce in your life time. That is why after a certain age it is best to start taking digestive enzymes with each meal. But, it is also wise to take digestive enzymes at any age.

Free Radicals

When you eat fruits, your cells digest or metabolize the fruit nutrients and leave behind free radicals. Antioxidants neutralize these free radicals. Free radicals attack internal cell material, cell membrane, and tissue, creating inflammation and all kinds of diseases. Antioxidants are the main natural remedy for preventing arteriosclerosis, coronary heart disease, senility, aging, cancer, cataracts and many other inflammatory diseases.

Vary the fruits you eat because they vary in the type of antioxidants and nutrients that they have. Antioxidant levels are reduced in fruits when they are exposed to excess heat, sun, cooking, pressure, and packaging. Eat fruits of different colors because they contain different types of antioxidants.

Eat fruits when they turn ripe to get the right alkaline minerals into your body. When they are green, they produce acid in your body and when they are overripe, they contain too much sugar.

Fruit Chemicals Not Discovered Yet

Fruits have hundreds of chemicals. Some are known and have been intensely studied. Others have yet to be discovered, and their purpose revealed. For this reason, it is best to eat a variety of fruits in the list given below, so that you can get the chemicals that can make you healthier, and that can cure any disease you might have.

7: Use Fruit-Vegetable Fiber to Fight Acids

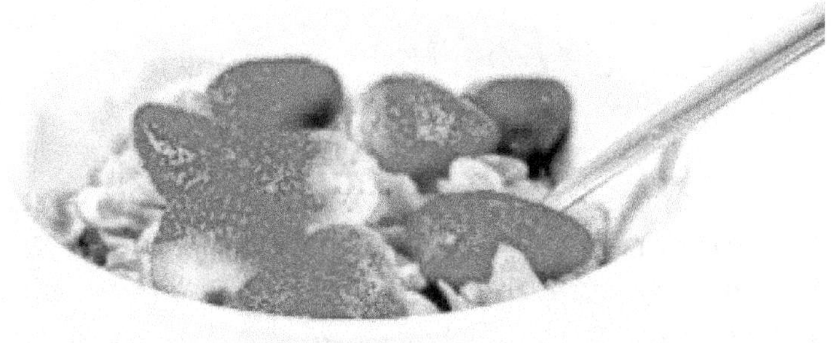

Fiber

All fruits contain fiber, some more than others. Fiber has many uses in the body. In the colon, it helps to prevent constipation, diverticulitis, hemorrhoids, and cancer and many other colon ills. Fiber pulls water into its structure as it goes through the intestines and colon, which softens the stool and makes it easier to pass through the colon.

If you don't eat enough fiber you will create an acid body. Without fiber, you will create a variety of illnesses. Being ill means you have an acid body. Eating fiber normalized and balances your body so that illness will not develop in your body.

If the food you have eaten does not have enough water, your stools will be hard and will have a difficult time moving through your colon. Then, if your stools sit in the colon too long, they will start to pull water out of your body, which can dehydrate you.

As fiber moves through the colon, it traps cholesterol, **acids**, toxins, carcinogens, estrogen, bile, **minerals**, and various un-digestible residues that come from the bile. Since fiber traps cholesterol and many other un-needed nutrients, they will not be reabsorbed by the colon walls. This prevents unwanted nutrients from getting back into your body to create body acids.

Fiber also traps sugar into its fibers, allowing sugar to slowly be absorbed by the small intestine. This helps diabetics to process complex carbohydrates without experiencing an overdose of blood sugar. Slowing down the absorption of sugar, allows the diabetic to decrease the diabetic drug dose.

Fiber also provides food for the good bacteria, probiotics, which gives your colon health.

It is recommended that you have at least 25 to 35 mg of fiber every day, and up to 35 mg and 40 mg is better. Most people are eating around 8 to 12 mg every day. When you move from eating 10 mg to 25 mg, you may develop stomach gas, since your body is not used to processing a large increase in fiber. Just start increasing your fiber use slowly every day for a couple of weeks until you reach 25 – 35 mg.

It is not recommended to eat an excess of fiber, over 35 to 40 mg per day, since fiber also tends to tie up minerals, thus preventing them from being absorbed into your body.

There are two types of fiber – soluble and insoluble. Soluble fiber dissolves in water and forms a gooey and sticky mass. One type of soluble fiber is pectin. Pectin is found on the outside of some fruits like apples and pears and some are contained inside the fruit.

Soluble Fiber

Soluble Fiber becomes gummy and viscous after it dissolves in water.

Soluble fiber has the ability to slow down digestion in the small intestine and prevent simple sugars from entering the bloodstream right away.

Because it absorbs water, soluble fiber softens and gives weight to fecal matter, and this makes fecal matter easier to pass through your colon.

Soluble fiber consists of pectin, gum, and mucilage. Pectin is found in carrots, apples, beets, cabbage, citrus fruits, and bananas. Gums and mucilage are found in oat bran, sesame seeds, oats, oatmeal, legumes, guar gum, and gum Arabic

Besides helping prevent constipation, soluble fiber provides the following benefits.

reduces the risk of heart disease

reduces the risk of gallstones

helps to remove toxic heavy metals and toxins from your colon

helps to prevent the toxic condition called appendicitis

regulates the movement of sugar into the bloodstream

helps to prevent hemorrhoids and fissures

lowers cholesterol

lowers absorption of fats in the intestines and most

importantly, helps prevent the overgrowth of bad bacteria in your colon.

Insoluble Fiber

Insoluble fiber does not dissolve in water and consists of cellulose, hemicellulose, and lignin. This type of fiber is extremely beneficial to your health. Because your body's enzymes cannot break down this fiber, like it does food, it remains in tack as it travels through your intestines and colon.

Insoluble fiber helps the fecal matter travel faster through the small intestine and your colon.

It provides bulk to your fecal matter. It makes your stools larger, softer, and stimulates peristaltic movement as it touches your colon walls.

Insoluble fiber, like soluble fiber, slows down digestion. It also slows down the absorption of protein, starch, and fat and can inhibit the action of digestive enzymes.

Insoluble fiber is found in vegetables, wheat, and wheat bran. This type of fiber is considered an anti-carcinogen and a digestive aid. It is credited with preventing colon cancer and many other colon diseases
.

Cellulose – Insoluble Fiber

Cellulose is a non-digestible carbohydrate which is found in the skins of fruits and vegetables – peas, green beans, carrots, broccoli, beets, brazil nuts, and lima beans.

Cellulose helps to remove cancer-causing toxins from your colon walls. It helps to prevent constipation, colitis, varicose veins, and hemorrhoids.

8: Use These Breakfast Ideas To Flush Out Acids

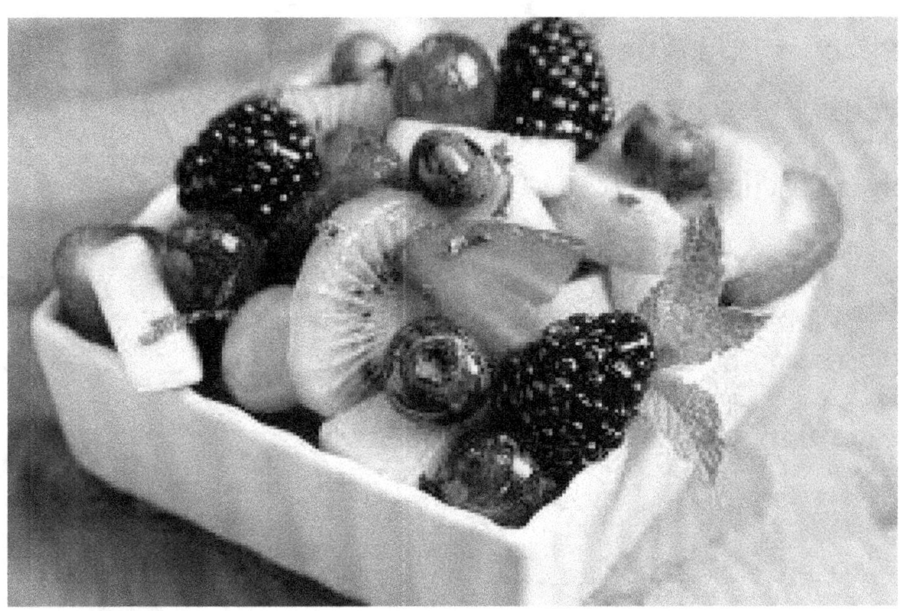

Breakfast

Here is a list of breakfast recipes that you can use, in the morning or any time you need a snack. These recipes can be used for cycle 1. Adjust the ingredients, for the number of people eating.

If you don't have some of the fruits in these recipes, use the ones you have.

Breakfast Pudding

5 large dates, pitted

1 apple, quartered and cored

1 large frozen banana

Several sections of orange, to taste

Place all ingredients into a blender. Add a bit of apple juice, to get the blender started.

Peaches and Blueberries with a Melon Bowl

4 peaches, peeled and cubed

1 cup blueberries

2 small cantaloupes, halved and seeded

With a spoon or knife, cut up the cantaloupe into small pieces and place them in a bowl, with the other fruits.

Pumpkin Applesauce Pudding

1 cup applesauce

¾ cup pumpkin puree

¼ cup raisins

Ground cinnamon, to taste

Ground nutmeg, to taste

Ground allspice, to taste

Combine all the ingredients in a bowl.

Fruit Salad

Bananas

Kiwis

Mandarin oranges

Pineapple

Apples

Fresh lemon or lime juice

Cut up the fruits and place them in a bowl. You can use other fruits that are in season.

Smoothies

Apple Berry Smoothie

1 cup apple juice

2 apples, peeled, quartered, and cored

½ cup fresh or frozen blueberries

½ cup blackberries

1 medium fresh or frozen banana

2 dates, pitted

Blend all ingredients, in a blender for one minute.

Banana Peach Drink

1 cup apple juice or orange juice

1 large fresh or frozen banana

2 ripe peaches, peeled, pitted, and cubed

Fresh strawberries

Blend all ingredients, in a blender for one minute.

Coconut Smoothie

1 cup regular or light coconut milk

1 tablespoon maca powder

1 tablespoon coconut oil

1 tablespoon ground flax seeds

1 teaspoon alcohol-free vanilla extract

¼ teaspoon almond extract

¼ teaspoon stevia powder

8-10 ice cubes

Blend all ingredients, in a blender for one minute.

Fruit Shake

8 ounces orange or apple juice

1 medium banana

½ cup frozen diced peaches (purchased or frozen

fresh)

Use any other fruit or combination of fruits that you like.

Strawberry Banana Smoothie

3 cups fresh strawberries

2 medium frozen bananas

1 cup fresh young coconut water

2 tablespoons raw hulled hemp seeds or ground

flax seeds

Blend all ingredients, in a blender for one minute.

Snacks between Meals

Avocado Dressing

4-6 ripe medium avocados

¼ cup fresh lime juice

¼ cup fresh lemon juice

½ teaspoon powdered garlic

1/3 cup olive oil

Water, as needed for consistency

Salt and pepper, to taste

Mix all ingredients in a bowl until avocados are smooth and not extra chunky.

Banana Avocado Snack

2 medium bananas, sliced

2 medium avocados, sliced

A squeeze of fresh lemon or lime juice

Salt to taste

Mix all ingredients in a bowl, until bananas and avocados are smooth and not extra chunky.

Guacamole

8-10 ripe medium avocados

2 tablespoons ground cumin

1 tablespoon garlic, minced

1 tablespoon ground coriander

¼ cup fresh lime juice

1/8 cup fresh lemon juice

2 large tomatoes, finely chopped

Mix all ingredients in a bowl, until avocados are smooth and not extra chunky. Cut this recipe down if you have fewer people to feed.

Tomato Basil Soup for Breakfast or Snack

> 5 large tomatoes (about 2 pounds), quartered
>
> 1 bunch fresh basil, chopped
>
> 2 cups vegetable broth
>
> 2 cloves garlic
>
> 2 teaspoon olive oil
>
> 2 tablespoons balsamic vinegar
>
> Salt and pepper, to taste
>
> Avocado chunks or sautéed eggplant, for garnish

You can eat this hot or cold. If you want to eat it hot, place all these ingredients into a pot and heat for 10 minutes.

Salads

California Morning Salad

> 1 somewhat firm avocado, diced
>
> 1 cucumber, diced
>
> 1 jalapeño chile pepper, sliced into thin rings
>
> 1 (3.8-ounce) can sliced olives
>
> Juice from 1 lemon
>
> Juice from 1 lime
>
> ¼ cup olive oil

Mix all ingredients into a bowl and toss.

Grapefruit with Avocado Salad

1 grapefruit, cut into segments and ¼ cup juice reserved

1 avocado, sliced or diced

¼ cup olive oil

¼- ½ teaspoon kosher salt

1 teaspoon Dijon mustard

Black pepper and black salt, to taste

Mix in a bowl and eat for breakfast or as a snack.

Banana Breakfast Pudding

1 medium ripe banana

6 dates, soaked in water for up to 30 minutes

2 to 3 peaches, pitted, or meat and water from 1 young coconut

2 teaspoon alcohol-free vanilla extract

1 teaspoon ground cinnamon

Agave nectar, to taste

Blend all Ingredients

9: Author and Resources

Rudy Silva is a natural nutritional consultant educated in the United States in Nutrition and Physics. He is a graduate of San Jose State University in California. He is the author of 40 other books on natural remedies. He has authored a newsletter in natural remedies for over 10 years.

Resource page

You can search google for the 40 other books I have written on natural healing.

If you need support or want to promote any of his e-books, please contact him at rss41@yahoo.com.

Give A Review

And, don't forget to give a review for this book at wherever you purchased it. It's not hard to give a review. It can be only a sentence or two. You don't have to leave a long review. A short review helps other people decide if they want to buy a book. So give a short review and give your thoughts to help other people and to help the author improve his book.

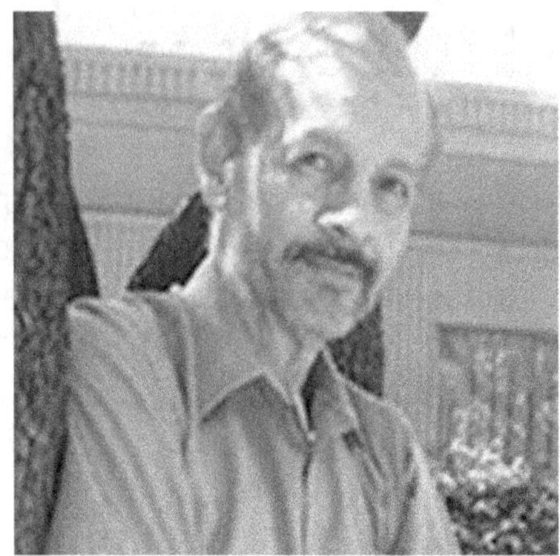

To you, for creating better health and more happiness,

Rudy S Silva

9 781725 004337